The Belief Road Map:

How to know yourself better and create personal philosophies to guide the way to the life of your dreams

Matt Gersper and Kaileen Sues

Happy Living Books
Independent Publishers
www.happyliving.

Printed in the United States of America

ISBN: 978-0-9972210-4-6

Disclaimer

Please note: this book and all content from Happy Living represents the personal opinions of Matt Gersper and Kaileen Elise Sues. Before making any changes to your diet or exercise routines, please consult a physician.

In memory of Coach Jim Sochor and Dr. Wayne Dyer, two men who's teaching of the Tao Te Ching has had a dramatic and very positive influence in shaping the philosophies of my life.

Dear reader,

I wish you every success in life that you can imagine!

Matt B. Gusper

Contents

Foreword

"You just gotta believe!"

Right?

Well, actually, something has to be created – a spark of sorts, before one can become AWARE.

After awareness can come reflection and a noticing. *The Belief Road Map* is one of those sparks.

I think of these sparks as "nudges" that we can give to one another. Kind of like, "Hey, how's that working out for ya?" That kind of nudge. Safe, harmless, but nonetheless powerful for what it can uncover and reveal.

A wise man once said that the best form of role modeling is exemplification. Matt Gersper has lived, and more importantly *is living*. I mean truly living as that role model for us all.

And *The Belief Road Map* is the guide he offers to help us truly live too. It will resonate with anyone who, like Matt, understands that Happy Living can be LIVED today. You *can* be happy right now, and your happiness can help and inspire others.

Sit back, enjoy and let *The Belief Road Map* be your guide for creating your best life right now.

Onward, upward.

James FitzGerald

Director of OPEX Fitness
2007 CrossFit Games Champion

Chapter 1 – Your Belief Road Map

"Live with intention. Walk to the edge. Listen hard. Practice wellness. Play with abandon. Laugh. Choose with no regret. Continue to learn. Appreciate your friends. Do what you love. Live as if this is all there is."
(Mary Anne Radmacher)

At one time or another, everyone has struggled with making decisions about their life. When you are standing at a crossroads and feeling under pressure, it is not the ideal moment for reflection. Knowing who you are, what you believe, and where you want to go in life takes time, effort and a strong sense of self. But big, life-altering moments often come out of nowhere and if you aren't prepared, you might find yourself making a decision that is fueled by "*musts*" and "*shoulds*" instead of based on the strong foundation of your personal beliefs.

Your Belief Road Map

If there is a part of you that feels stuck, held back by your job, friends, family, the city you live in, or another factor that seems beyond your control, you are not alone. People everywhere move along in life without stoking the fires of their dreams or breathing life into their inner desires. Doing what you think society, your parents, partner, or community wants you to do will only keep you feeling stuck and held back. The way to feel alive again is to learn about your inner beliefs and use those as your road map to the life of your dreams.

For many of us, life was simple when we were young. If we were lucky, we had our basic needs met and were able to focus on the important things – exploring, playing, laughing, making friends, and having fun. Childhood is filled with wonderful moments, but it is also a time when our connection to who we truly are inside starts to weaken from the demands of society. Along the way, people tell us what we should do and who we should become. Many of us lose the ability to listen to our intuition and inner guidance, and instead are always looking to others for direction.

If you feel like you have been wandering through life following a formula – school to work to family to retirement to death – but have not found true fulfillment in the journey so far, perhaps it is time to change. Whether you are just starting on your path of personal development or have spent years working on yourself, now is the time to begin using your inner compass. It is the only way to find the fulfillment you are seeking.

For a moment, think about the process of taking a vacation or planning a trip. First, you start with research and decide on a destination that excites or intrigues you. Then you book a flight or get driving directions. Next, you think about where you would like to stay and what you want to do when you get there. Obvious, right? Most people don't just show up at the airport and step onto the first plane they see, and yet many of us wander through life without any clear direction in mind. Similar to this example, life is also a journey that requires thoughtful planning. You might truly desire a tranquil town, but end up in a very busy city instead. Or perhaps you have always wanted to live abroad, but find yourself still in the hometown where you were born. Without a Belief Road Map in place, there's no telling where you might end up.

When you know who you are and what you believe, you will start living with the most powerful inner compass imaginable. You will discover opportunities suited to your skills and strengths, you will meet people who you connect with on a deeper level, and you will start to believe in yourself and your dreams. In short, you will begin to walk through life with purpose.

Discover Your True Beliefs

Discovering your true beliefs and then living by them is not an easy process. First, it takes time and effort to get to the heart of who you are as a person and how you want to live in the world. You might have to throw away beliefs that no longer serve you and redefine your dreams to align them with your heart. You will need to have the courage to be honest with yourself and the willingness to act in alignment with your truth. If this were a simple and straightforward path, everyone in the world would be successful, happy, and filled with peace. Sometimes it seems much easier to let others tell you where to go, and of course, we were all taught to do this as children because it suited others along the way. There's no judgment in that – everyone is doing the best they can with what they know. But that was then and this is now. It is important to remember that you have the choice of whether to use someone else's Belief Road Map or to make your own.

Identify Your Priorities

Identifying your priorities and using your beliefs to create personal philosophies is the cure to wandering aimlessly through life. First, you select a particular topic, like health or fitness, and then dive deep into your beliefs about why it is important to you, what it means to you, and what kind of role you want it to play in your life. Through this process you will gain the power to set up your life, and to make decisions, in alignment with your inner wisdom. Without this type of self-inquiry, you might have a sense that fitness is important to you, but it will be much easier to put exercise on the backburner for other things that are less meaningful. Fitness is only one example, but being disconnected from our beliefs, and therefore our inner compass, is how we lose our way. The magical thing is, you can always get back on track by taking the time to look inward and find your true north. Give yourself permission to stop following the formula of *"shoulds"* in your head. Instead, start listening to your heart and following your dreams. *The Belief Road Map* will show you how.

Meet Matt Gersper

This book is based on the life experience, personal study, and process of turning inspiration into action created by Matt Gersper. Together with his daughter, Kaileen Elise Sues, Matt launched his health and wellness company, Happy Living, in 2014 with one mission in mind: to improve the health and wellbeing of the world, one person at a time.

As a young boy, Matt dreamt of becoming a professional football player. Despite being small for his age, he trained hard and believed with every fiber of his being that he would one day reach his goal. Matt ended up growing into a strong safety, playing for his college football team, the UC Davis Aggies, and trying out for three professional football teams.

When it became clear that he would just fall short of that dream, Matt directed his tenacity and work ethic towards being successful in business. He climbed the corporate ladder for several years until he was fired over a disagreement with the management. While it was a blow to his ego, he used the experience of getting fired as an opportunity to buy an existing global trade business, which he purchased for $1.5 million and sold for $42 million ten years later.

After the successful sale of his business in 2014, he embarked on his next adventure and followed his heart to start Happy Living, a new company that would give back to the world. Through every step of his journey, Matt has relied on self-reflection, goal setting, and listening to his heart. This book shares his personal philosophies on life. And it's not all about the good stuff – even in the midst of failures like being cut from several professional football training camps, getting fired from an impressive executive position, and personal struggles like facing divorce after 24 years of marriage, Matt's Belief Road Map has lit the path for new discoveries and adventures. You too can find the same stable, solid base, which will support you through whatever life brings to you.

Now at the age of 54, Matt believes that a better self and a more fulfilled, joyful life is possible right now, today, and every day for the rest of his life. It is his hope that this book will empower you to believe the same about yourself and your precious, unique life as well.

How to Use This Book

You can read *The Belief Road Map* for pure inspiration and to get new ideas for living a happy and fulfilling life. You can breeze through it and then let the parts that resonate with you settle in. Or you can use it as a workbook to craft your own philosophies on life, reading it slowly and taking time to reflect on each piece that speaks to you. You might want to journal about your thoughts as you go along, or talk with a friend, loved one or mentor. You could also reflect on your discoveries during exercise, meditation, or prayer.

However you approach it, *The Belief Road Map* is intended to provide you with the tools you need to reveal your true self and help you gain clarity on what's most important to you. Creating your personal philosophies will empower you to make decisions that are true to your heart. Using your beliefs as a road map will help you persevere in the face of adversity and give you the courage to follow your dreams. Do not let life pass by without discovering who you really are and what you truly believe. Be confident in your decisions. Believe in yourself. Know where you want to go and how to get there. Go after your dreams! And let your Belief Road Map be your guide.

Are you ready to begin your life's next adventure? Let's get started.

Chapter 2 – The Power of Reflection

"The meaning of life is to give life meaning."
(Ken Hudgins)

"Who am I?" is both a very simple and complex question to answer. You probably have a quick response during dinner party conversations that includes your name, job, and details about where you are from. Family and close friends know a different 'you' with inside jokes and stories from your past. But even deeper, tucked within your heart, you have the true answer that encompasses every dream and secret desire, all of your passions and stories, fears, truths, and lies. This answer to the question, "Who am I?" is the essence of you and the core of what drives your beliefs. This is the 'you' we are aiming to connect with throughout this book.

So, how do you connect to your truest, most fundamental 'you'? Well, reflection is a powerful tool for answering the key question, "Who am I?" and unlocking your true beliefs.

What is Reflection?

Reflection is the process of spending time in thought, contemplation, or meditation on everything from your personal memories to the current trends unfolding around you, as well as things that have happened throughout history. Reflection can help you make new connections between old experiences and new situations. Something that may not have seemed relevant or noteworthy at the time can spark great insight when viewed through the lens of reflection. As Soren Kierkegaard once said, "Life can only be understood backwards; but it must be lived forwards."

Reflection is most effective when the mind is quiet and clear of distraction. It can be hard to find the time and space for true, meaningful contemplation in the midst of our busy lives. Constant multitasking, rushing from one meeting to the next, and eating dinner in front of the TV are hallmarks of most people's everyday lives. So if reflection is important to you, there are some steps you can take in order to make the time and space for it to happen. From our years of personal experience, we promise it will be worth your while! In addition to being a profound undertaking in itself, reflection will enrich all the fun, busy, and packed-full parts of your life too.

Rather than waiting for the ideal moment for reflection (which, in your busy schedule, may simply never come!), begin to carve out chunks of time for it. For example, you might try to wake up 30 minutes earlier and start your day with journaling. Or, you can spend time during your lunch break in quiet contemplation. You can even utilize things that are already part of your day-to-day activity, like showering and exercise, and make those your times for reflection. Matt likes to reflect while on long hikes, out paddle boarding, and during meditation.

Taking Time to Know Yourself

Knowing yourself is a lifelong process. Just like any other relationship, you cannot spend 15 minutes with yourself and know everything there is to know about your beliefs, dreams, and desires. But all journeys are traveled one step at a time, so as you start this process remember to be kind and patient with yourself. You could also make a commitment to yourself to spend a few minutes in reflection whenever you remember. Part of you might think you can always "do it later," but we encourage you to seize the time when you have it. And please don't get down on yourself if you miss one of your reflection sessions. The fact that you are doing this work is wonderful, period – and it really can be easy and fun.

Try These Reflection Techniques

There are many ways to reflect on your life. One interesting activity is to look at how you spend your time, money, and attention. Look at every single financial transaction for the past month. Review your calendar carefully, taking note of your meetings and appointments. How did you spend your downtime? Think about where you were and whom you were with. These are clues to your current priorities.

And how do you tell whether your current priorities are in line with your true self? By noticing how you feel about them. If you are elated with how you've been spending your time and money, then it's likely that your actions are in alignment with your true desires. If you feel frustrated or disappointed, think about why that might be. Were you with someone who puts you down, however subtly? Or did you feel pressure to spend that money to "keep up with the neighbors" or to receive approval from outside yourself? Once you've completed the exercise, take a moment to reflect on the process too. How did it make you feel? Did some painful feelings come up or did you find a sense of power in gaining new insight? What sort of information have you gathered about where you are, or are not, in alignment with your true self?

In his book *Halftime: Moving from Success to Significance*, Bob Buford suggests that readers create a mission statement for their lives and write their own epitaph. Exercises like these are a prime opportunity for reflection. What is your legacy and how do you want to be remembered? What is your mission in life and what kind of impact do you want to leave on the world?

Let Your Inner Wisdom Guide You

Answering questions like these can help uncover your inner beliefs and most precious dreams. By hearing your own answers, you'll be more in touch with your inner wisdom, and you will be able to let it guide you. Also, if you find it challenging to think about yourself in a positive, kind way during this exercise, take a few deep breaths and tell yourself that you're doing great. Acknowledging fear or anxiety through this process is actually your route to self-esteem and empowerment, so well done and keep at it!

Giving yourself the time and space to reflect on life will help you develop a stronger sense of self. So many of us let the outside influences of news, social media, family, friends, and co-workers cloud our judgment. But in truth, external opinions should never hold more power than what is within our heart and mind. That's not to say there isn't value in seeking knowledge! There are many topics you might find interesting that will require research and study in order to form your personal beliefs. When you are intrigued by something, and the idea of looking into it fills you with excitement that is your inner wisdom speaking up. Follow that inner wisdom and you will connect with your beliefs.

Reflection Brings Connections

As you use the power of reflection, you might find you're making connections and having revelations without even trying. Things you never noticed before will come to the forefront, and life will bring you more of what you focus on. For example, you might start to study cooking because it brings you joy, and then you notice that you have a friend or co-worker who can teach you some things in the kitchen. By paying attention to your thoughts and feelings, you are cultivating a sense of curiosity about the world, while strengthening your relationship with yourself.

Reflection Brings Awareness

"I did then what I knew how to do. Now that I know better, I do better."
(Maya Angelou)

Without self-reflection, we go through our daily lives pulled along by myriad influences. At times, there might be a sense of discomfort that comes from within. Without an inner compass, it is impossible to understand what doesn't resonate with our hearts, or how we can find what does. Reflection gives us the power to understand ourselves. We can begin to know why we say what we say, why we do what we do, and why we are who we are. We can start knowing better and doing better.

Reflection gives us the knowledge to change course when necessary. It also gives us the insight to stop trying to constantly fix, change, and improve upon things (which our busy minds love to do) and instead appreciate all we are and all we have. Knowing your core beliefs – what is most important to you and the things that bring you joy – is how you start to live by your Belief Road Map.

What will knowing better and doing better look like? For some, it might be a complete life transformation. You might need to do something big like move across country, go back to school, or start a business. For others, it will be a series of subtle, internal shifts that are impossible to recognize from the outside – apart from by the beaming smile on your face, your relaxed, easy-going energy, and your joyful engagement with friends and family, of course! Your personality, who you are, and where you are in life will influence what it means to live by your Belief Road Map. We'll be exploring this more in the following chapters.

Then, when you have a sense of your personal beliefs, we will share Matt's personal philosophies, which act as mile markers on his own Belief Road Map. These philosophies draw on his life experience, years of study, and hours of reflection. Each one is an essay about his beliefs on a particular topic of priority in his life, including, love, adventure, and significance. It is our humble hope that they will inspire you with even more ideas for your own personal Belief Road Map

<u>Chapter 3 – Priorities Guide the Way</u>

So, how do you uncover the beliefs that will guide the way to the life of your dreams? The best way to begin is by defining your priorities.

In the previous chapter, you used the power of reflection to examine how you feel about where you are and what you're doing in your life right now. So, ask yourself, "What feels good and what doesn't? What are my true priorities?" A short list of what's most important might come to mind automatically. Or you could need more time to reflect on what you want to make a priority in your life. In quiet and solitude, through journaling or meditation, you might discover things you hadn't realized were important to you.

Those Pesky "*Shoulds*"

Before we talk anymore about priorities, we want to ask if there are things in your life that feel like they "*should*" be priorities? Everyone has external pressures and influences that make us feel like we "*should*" be doing this or that, which is why it is critical to differentiate between the obligations and priorities in our lives. Paying the mortgage or taxes are obligations, but being able to donate to charity might be a priority. Priorities, obligations, and "*shoulds*" play different roles in our lives and we ought to treat them differently too.

Your Dreams and Goals

Think for a minute about your dreams and goals. Where do you want to go in life? Who do you want to be? It does not matter if you are 18, 88, or somewhere in between, we all have inner desires and dreams. Imagine your ideal life 10 years from now. Where do you live, how do you spend your time, who are you with, and how does your life make you feel? Now think back to your priorities. How are they reflected in your dreams and your ideal scenario? If you find parallels and correlations, then your priorities are in alignment with your beliefs.

For example, if your dream is to become an Olympic swimmer, your priorities might include training, eating healthy, getting enough rest, and improving your mental stamina. If your dream is to become a best-selling author, your priorities might be to write, research, brainstorm ideas, and read the works of authors you admire. If your dream is to be a good role model for your children or younger siblings, your priorities might be to act in alignment with your beliefs, pursue your dreams, and treat your family with generosity and kindness.

When your priorities are in alignment with your goals and beliefs, they will make you feel empowered and strong, happy and at peace. Just think, if you were able to live by these priorities each week, month, year and decade, your life would be fulfilling and fun! Once you know your priorities and write them down for easy reference, living by them becomes a lot more possible. Your actions and decisions can come from a place of clarity and conviction. While it might not always be easy to live by your priorities and beliefs, you will have the assurance that you are coming from a place of personal power. Instead of doing things because you "should," you will do them because you have chosen them and made them a priority in your life.

You are already doing a bunch of things every day. This process of identifying your priorities helps you spend as little time as necessary on the "*shoulds*" and obligations. When you start living by your priorities, you will automatically start clearing time and space for the things that matter most to you. Once you begin to live in harmony with your core beliefs and priorities, the "*shoulds*" in your life will grab your attention less often. You might even find creative ways to make them a bit more fun and fulfilling!

In the next chapter, we will outline what we like to call the Seven Foundations of Health. These are what we consider to be the priorities for living a healthy, abundant, and happy life. You might find some similarities between your priorities and ours, and if one resonates that you hadn't thought of, please do add it to your list. Just as you are a completely unique individual, your priorities will be very personal to you too.

Chapter 4 – The Seven Foundations of Health

"Health is a state of complete harmony of the body, mind and spirit."
(B.K.S. Iyengar)

Health is more than living in a body that is free from disease. Rather, health is a daily practice, a journey, and relationship – with one's self, others, and the world. When we founded our company, Happy Living, we made it our mission to improve the health and wellbeing of the world, one person at a time. This is both a very ambitious and attainable goal. In one respect, we have set out to change the world, and at the same time, we are simply focused on each individual person we help. To work toward our mission, we have defined our priorities and what health means to us.

As you read through this next section, we encourage you to think about your personal definitions of health and wellness. How do your priorities support or influence your beliefs about what it means to be healthy? We offer our Seven Foundations of Health as an example and so that you can gather inspiration if they resonate with you.

Our Seven Foundations of Health are:

- Physical Fitness

- Mental Fitness

- Spiritual Fitness

- Financial Fitness

- Love

- Adventure

- Significance

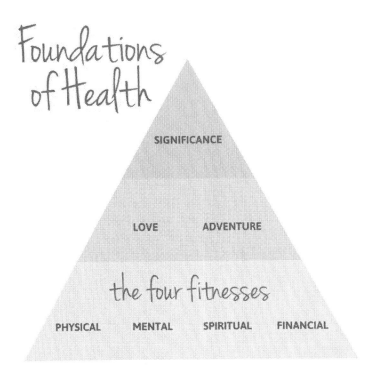

happyliving.com

We think of these Seven Foundations of Health as a pyramid with the four "fitnesses" at the base. In the busy world we live in, we believe it is more important than ever to take personal accountability for health. Dedicating time, effort, and energy to each of the four fitnesses is a crucial part of our journey.

The Four Fitnesses

Physical Fitness is usually what comes to mind first when thinking about health. Physical fitness includes exercise, nutrition, hydration and sleep, as well as important health maintenance like doctor's visits, diagnostics, and blood work.

Mental Fitness is commonly referred to as mental health. Even though it's within the mind and not as tangible as physical fitness, it is just as vital. In addition to caring for mental illness, mental fitness includes reading, meditation and reflection, goal setting, creativity, lifelong learning, and the pursuit of hobbies.

Spiritual Fitness is the connection between our inner self and something greater. It can be faith-based, found through meditation, or observed through science. It may be cultivated within a community or alone, and it is something we can always come back to no matter how much time has passed.

Financial Fitness is being able to financially provide for yourself and others. It includes living within your means, in alignment with your priorities, and in a way that does not put financial strain on savings. It is being informed and educated about finances, as well as giving to charity and causes – when possible and when it resonates with your heart. While it is important to save and make wise investment decisions, we believe it is also important to spend the money we earn with happiness and pride.

Love and Adventure

The next two elements in the Seven Foundations of Health are love and adventure, which create the center of the pyramid.

Love is essential to a healthy and meaningful life. Love gives substance to relationships. Love is what pushes us to pursue our passions. Love breathes peace into quiet moments. Love helps us persevere through tough times. Self-love, or the relationship we have with ourselves, is just as important to happy living as loving others. Without self-love, we cannot offer our best to those around us or to the work we do. Love provides us with purpose, happiness, and joy. As Henry Drummond once said, "You will find as you look back upon your life that the moments when you have truly lived are the moments when you have done things in the spirit of love."

Adventure is embarking on uncharted territory and welcoming new discoveries. Adventure is not just about being extreme, although the possibility of danger might excite your daring side. Adventure can happen close to home or far away, it can be a state of mind or an epic getaway. Maintaining a practice of adventure is vital to longevity. If you really want to do something, but it scares you a little, that's usually a good sign!

Significance

At the peak of the pyramid lies significance. Significance is a key to happiness and wellbeing. The pursuit of significance adds meaning to life. Significance is a habit of prioritizing those things that are most important to you. Significance is dedicating your time, work, resources, and life to something of great personal meaning. Your "something significant" can be anything from a tangible goal to the legacy you leave behind. It does not matter where you begin. Focusing on gratitude, acting with purpose, and pursuing your dreams are all ways to practice significance. A deep sense of satisfaction or feeling of being honored to be part of an activity, relationship, or event is a sign that it holds great significance for you.

Happy, healthy living is not a destination or a point to work towards. It is a consistent practice of choice, discipline and good habits… that work for you. These Seven Foundations of Health are at the heart of our work at Happy Living. In the next chapter, we're going to give a deeper look at your priorities and beliefs and then begin the process of creating your personal philosophies.

Chapter 5 – Your Personal Philosophies

Now that you have used the power of reflection to reveal your beliefs and priorities, have you noticed anything different? Has your outlook on life shifted? Has your decision-making process changed? Are your choices slightly different than before? Maybe you've listened to your heart and said no to someone rather than taking on "just one more" project? Perhaps you've decided that you'd rather save and plan for that expensive vacation rather than put it on a credit card? These are just a couple of examples – there is no right or wrong here, just what is in line with your inner wisdom.

Defining Your Personal Philosophies

When you reflected on your beliefs and priorities, did you notice discrepancies or things you want to change? Taking the next step to define your personal philosophies will help bring clarity. Personal philosophies are the guiding principles of your beliefs and the road map to the life of your dreams. Your philosophies are definitions of what you think, want, need, and hope for your specific priorities. In the next several chapters, we will share Matt's personal philosophies, some of which are based on Happy Living's Seven Foundations of Health.

Matt's philosophies are based on his life experience, from his start as a small boy with dreams of being a professional football player, to his successful career as an entrepreneur and business owner. With every step, Matt has used his personal philosophies as the foundation for a road map to his dreams. His philosophies are the definition and guiding force of his daily pursuit of personal improvement.

Inspired by the book *Halftime* by Bob Buford, Matt defined the one big thing that is most important in his life, as well as his epitaph and mission. While these exercises were extremely challenging and took some time to complete, Matt found them to be invigorating and helpful in defining his personal philosophies.

Matt's "One Big Thing," Epitaph, and Mission

Matt's "one big thing" is The Tao. The Tao literally means "the Way."

According to *The Untethered Soul* by Michael A. Singer, Lao Tzu's ancient teachings are the guiding philosophy of life, in eighty-one short verses. Matt believes his daily study of Lao Tzu's *Tao Te Ching*, along with his practice of the Tao's philosophies, are his path to becoming all he is capable of in this lifetime.

His epitaph is, "My life is my mission," because the phrase represents an attitude of allowing rather than interfering, of acting rather than advising. Instead of presuming to know the best route for another's journey, Matt believes he can help others by sharing what he is doing on his.

Matt's mission for his life is the same as ours at Happy Living: to improve the health and wellbeing of the world, one person at a time. This mission is his way of giving back to the world and inspiring others to become all they are capable of with the unique gifts they have been given.

Matt's "one big thing," epitaph and mission have influenced his personal philosophies. As you read through them, you can gather examples of how this process might go best for you. Feel free to borrow inspiration from his philosophies… or even identify things with which you disagree.

Refining Your Priorities

Before reading on, you might want to think about which of your priorities could benefit from further thought, reflection, and definition. And maybe feel out what's still missing from your list. What role do your priorities play on the road to your dreams? How can your priorities help you achieve your life's mission? Well, your priorities will be at the heart of your personal philosophies.

You might also want to reflect on what type of things you want to include in your philosophies. Is there a timeframe, frequency, or duration that is relevant? Are your philosophies something you will practice on your own or as part of a wider community? Why are your philosophies important to you? How are they part of your life? What kinds of practices or habits will you employ to ensure your priorities *remain* important to you?

Creating Your Personal Philosophies

Finally, another thing to consider is how you will create your personal philosophies. You might find that writing your priorities, personal philosophies, and beliefs out in a journal or on your computer is a therapeutic and helpful practice. Or, you might prefer to create a bulleted list, take notes on post-its, or make a visual collage that represents your beliefs. You could try all of these or some other variation. The key is to get your inner reflections out of your mind and into your world – the form, digital or otherwise, does not matter.

Make sure to keep your philosophies in an accessible place. We have found that it's important to revisit our personal philosophies on a regular basis. So do what you can to make them part of your everyday life. You might want to try placing them somewhere you will see often, or you could even ask a friend or family member to support you by reminding you to spend time working with your philosophies.

If now is a good time for you, get started on your philosophies immediately. Or you can read on and gather some inspiration from Matt's philosophies in the chapters that follow, and then compose your own from there. However you proceed, we are right with you, appreciating your commitment to bringing change, happiness, and harmony into your life.

Chapter 6 – My Philosophy for Happy Living

The first of Matt's philosophies sets out his perspective on what it means to live a fulfilling and happy life. His philosophy on happy living is over-arching and includes the principles that guide him and the rest of his philosophies. So, in the following chapters, we're going to let Matt take the floor, to share his first-hand personal experiences and discoveries with you.

> "The great vessel is slow to mature."
> (Lao Tzu)

My philosophy for healthy, happy living focuses on my desire to become a fully realized and optimized person, by my own definitions. Developing this philosophy has been 54 years in the making — and it will continue to be a lifelong endeavor. My philosophy for happy living has been tested through trials, tribulations, failures, and successes. I have played and experimented with life to see what works for me. This is what I've learned so far…

It all begins with gratitude. I work hard, believe in myself, and try my best to overcome the challenges life brings. Perhaps my biggest life lesson has been to shift my focus from what I want, to having gratitude for what I have and where I am at the moment – to live each day like nothing is missing. I start most mornings with this simple expression of gratitude:

I am alive.

I am loved.

I am in love.

Creating a healthy, happy life takes practice and intention. Lifelong learning inspires me to continuously develop new ideas and skills. Lifelong reflection and reassessment of my priorities helps me stay focused on what's truly important.

I know that it doesn't matter how fast I go, it only matters that I keep moving forward. I have learned to be patient and diligent, to be self-supportive, and to give myself time to progress in a purposeful direction with consistency and daily practice.

I let inspiration lead the way. I am at my happiest when I am listening to my heart. I have grown to trust my heart because it knows where my happiness lies. When a thought or an idea inspires me, I can feel it in my body. I pay attention to that sensation.

When an idea strikes me, I make sure it's relevant for me. I compare it to my top priorities from my practices of reflection and reassessment. This helps me separate inspirational ideas that I want to act on from really cool ones that I just want to acknowledge and then leave alone.

For example, inspiration struck when I was speaking at a conference and it was from that moment that I decided to write my first book. Around the same time, I also saw a super cool seaplane land on the lake in front of my home. I thought to myself, "Wouldn't it be great to own a seaplane!?"

I brought in my priorities as filters for both of these ideas. After thinking about how each related to what's most important to me, the result was that I acknowledged the seaplane as cool, and turned my focus back to writing.

I try to spend my time on things that are inspiring and fit my priorities, and drop whatever else I possibly can. This is a very precise and systematic approach, I know, and I don't think that's a bad thing. There is powerful energy in maintaining order.

> "Maintaining order rather than correcting disorder is the ultimate principle of wisdom. To cure disease after it has appeared is like digging a well when one feels thirsty, or forging weapons after the war has already begun."
> (Nei Jing)

I couldn't agree more. I have found through my life experience that it is much easier to maintain order than to correct disorder. I am happiest when I live my life in an orderly way. When things get disorderly, it takes lots of extra energy to get them back on track.

In his excellent book, *The Untethered Soul*, Michael A. Singer explains the secret of maintaining order with simple, almost rhetorical, questions about the Tao Te Ching:

> "Is it good for a person to eat sometimes? Yes, obviously it is. Is it good for a person to eat all the time? No, of course not. Somewhere in between, you passed over the Tao.
>
> Is it good to fast periodically? Yes. Is it good to never eat? No.
>
> The pendulum can swing all the way from gorging yourself to death, to starving yourself to death. Those are the two extremes of the pendulum: the yin and the yang, expansion and contraction, nondoing and doing.
>
> Everything has two extremes. Everything has gradations of this pendulum swing. If you go to the extremes you cannot survive."

Life has taught me that I have more energy and I am happier when I focus on my priorities, maintain order in my life, and avoid extremes.

Every life is full of obstacles, failures, and setbacks. Mine is no exception. I simply try to do the right thing. When I slip up, I have learned to forgive myself quickly, without judgment, get back up, and get back at it.

Meaningful work fosters happiness within. I believe I was made to work and I know I am happiest when I'm engaged in meaningful work. In addition to cultivating a sense of purpose, work provides the means to be responsible.

In my life, work has given me the ability to be responsible for myself, to care for my family, and give to others. Work has also provided me with countless hours of inspiration and learning. Dedicating myself to meaningful work has shown me that I can overcome challenges and create the life I want.

I am most fulfilled when I'm engaged in creative work, producing something that makes a contribution to society, and doing so in connection with my family, friends and community.

My philosophy for happy living is built on the concepts of gratitude, inspiration, maintaining order, and doing work that is meaningful. Living by this philosophy is the groundwork for my belief that a better self is always possible – today, tomorrow, every day, and for the rest of our time on this planet.

Chapter 7 – My Philosophy for Physical Fitness

My next two philosophies focus on the first of the four fitnesses: physical fitness. Through a lifetime of research and practice, I have cultivated daily practices for my diet and exercise regime that are personalized and in alignment with my priorities and lifelong goals.

> "Exercise is King. Nutrition is Queen. Put them together and you've got a kingdom."
> (Jack LaLanne)

Physical fitness is the cornerstone of the Seven Foundations of Health. A cornerstone is the first stone in the building of a structure. In the case of your health and happiness, it is the most important stone. Without it, the entire structure crumbles. The way I see it, you can't be much good to anyone or anything without your health.

Diet

What I have learned is that physical fitness is comprised of both exercise and nutrition. Jack LaLanne was a personal trainer and fitness expert who was way out in front with this knowledge. He believed, "Every human being can attain maximum body health and fitness if they will practice moderation, eat the most natural foods, and exercise on a regular basis."

While committing to consistent, lifelong exercise has come naturally for me, creating a healthy nutritional practice has not. For most of my adult life, I did not think or care much about food. As long as I maintained a weight that felt comfortable, I ate as I pleased. If my weight increased, I ate less. That was my "nutritional practice." I took better care of my car than my body. I fueled my car with premium gasoline and fed my body with junk. In 2010, I had a cholesterol scare that motivated me to change my ways. I began to think about physical health as not just exercise, but also nutrition. Since then, I have learned that I cannot exercise my way out of a bad diet.

There are a few elements to my nutritional philosophy that I have found work best for me. I have tweaked and adjusted these ideas through personal study, experimentation, and measuring my results.

My diet in a nutshell: eat real food with a focus on reducing inflammation.

My journey to better nutrition began in the summer of 2013. Inspired by the book *Wheat Belly* by William Davis, MD, my wife and I made the decision to eliminate wheat and other grains from our diet. I wasn't too concerned about the difficulty of our decision until I realized that no grains also meant no beer! Giving up my lifelong love for beer seemed like a colossal commitment.

However, the very first day of my "wheat-free and beer-free" diet, I felt better. The bloating and stomach gas that had become normal for me began to dissipate. Over the next thirty days, I stuck to the diet and continued to feel better and better.

Since then I have learned that a diet high in wheat, sugar, bad fats, toxic chemicals, and additives causes inflammation at the cellular level. When this happens, nutrients cannot get into our cells to create energy and antioxidants, and toxins can't get out. Inflammation and cellular damage can make us sick, and can speed up the aging process. On the other hand, reducing systemic inflammation restores the body's ability to function properly and helps maintain optimal health.

I have modified my diet to eliminate (or reduce) foods that damage my health and replace them with those which nourish my body so it functions the way it was designed.

Dr. David Perlmutter, renowned neurologist and author of *Grain Brain*, has some simple advice for helping you make good food choices. He says, "If it can go bad, it's good for you. If it stays good, it's bad for you."

I follow the dietary guidelines outlined in *Grain Brain* by fueling my body with healthy fats, proteins, and vegetables, and limiting carbohydrates. I buy organic foods when possible and shop at the local farmers' market frequently. When I am grocery shopping, I focus on the perimeter of the store where the natural and fresh foods are located.

Additionally, I believe in the Japanese teaching of *hara hachi bu*, which instructs people to eat until they are 80 percent full. This is a simple and beautiful concept that resonates with me. It's a relatively new addition to my daily practice that I am working to master.

I cannot get all the essential nutrients my body needs from food alone, so I supplement my diet with products specifically designed to promote healthy aging and longevity. My daily supplements include Coenzyme Q-10, Resveratrol, Omega-3 Fatty Acids, brain-boosting nutrients, melatonin, and a blend designed to offer support for aging.

I also do a monthly detox with a full day cleanse to support my body's natural ability to remove toxins and impurities. Throughout the day, I drink water along with four servings of a cleansing mixture. I do not eat food of any kind, nor do I drink any alcohol on cleansing day. However, I do permit myself to enjoy my cherished morning coffee.

I use my monthly cleansing day to focus on spirituality. I slow my daily pace, schedule less, and meditate more. I spend time in nature with longer, slower hikes through the woods. I dedicate time to reflection, giving appreciation to all I have, and thinking deeply about what I want to create with the rest of my life.

Several measurements help me track the progress of my fitness, inside and out:

- Body weight: I record my weight each month after my cleanse day

- Resting heart rate: Each month, I use a heart rate monitor to measure my resting heart rate for three mornings in a row and then calculate the 3-day average

- Cholesterol: I record my cholesterol markers twice a year, using a web-based service to order blood work without having to visit my primary care physician

Since I committed to my nutritional philosophy, I have noticed that I rarely feel hungry. My persistent sniffles and runny nose have disappeared. The constant bloated feeling is gone and my stomach has flattened. Being healthier makes me feel great... and sometimes that is the best measurement of all!

Exercise

My philosophy for lifelong exercise has been more than forty years in the making. From my years as a young boy playing in the neighborhood to my pursuit of professional football as a career, exercising is as much a part of my daily life as brushing my teeth. Like personal hygiene, I make it a non-negotiable activity. I just do it, whether I feel like it or not... and I almost always feel better after.

Consistent exercise is a personal productivity booster. It makes me stronger, healthier, and happier. I think of my physical fitness as fuel – it creates energy to support the other Foundations of Health: mental fitness, spiritual fitness, financial fitness, love, adventure, and significance. I find that committing to consistent, lifelong exercise comes naturally. I have sometimes wondered why this comes easy for me when so many other people struggle with it. I believe it is because of several techniques and tactics I use on a daily basis.

"It doesn't matter how fast you go, as long as you don't stop." (Confucius)

1. Do what you enjoy.

In order to get in shape and maintain fitness, you have to move. That can mean hiking, swimming, playing a sport, gardening, rowing, yoga, Pilates, etc. Try different activities and identify the ones you like and have fun doing.

2. Do it regularly.

I make an effort to do some form of exercise nearly every day, and plan to keep doing so for the rest of my life.

3. Don't give it back.

It takes work and dedication to get in shape. Once you reach a certain level of fitness, determine that you will not give it back. I learned long ago that we lose fitness three times faster than we gain it. So if you take a week off, you lose three weeks. It's not worth it!

4. Do it slowly.

Be careful and take your time getting into shape. Then, when you've reached a level you're happy with, and only then, think about staying in shape for life. A common mistake people make is starting too fast and going too hard. Another is expecting immediate results even when it took years to get out of shape. Inevitably they get injured, or they cannot sustain the pace they have set, or they don't meet the high expectations they created for themselves – and they give up.

I do my best to lighten up, but I never give up. I show up and don't quit. I go easy, go often and keep going every day. As Lao Tzu proclaimed more than 2,500 years ago, "The journey of a thousand miles begins with a single step."

Chapter 8 – My Philosophy for Mental Fitness

In the Seven Foundations of Health, mental fitness follows physical fitness. My philosophy on mental fitness outlines the ways in which I care for one of my most important assets, my mind.

> "The brain is transforming itself constantly. Just as you cannot step into a river in the same place twice, you can't step into the brain in the same place twice. Both are flowing. The brain is a process, not a thing; a verb, not a noun."
>
> (*Super Brain* by Deepak Chopra, MD and Rudolph E. Tanzi, PhD)

I grew up believing that the neural pathways of my brain were fixed and immutable. Science told us brain cells died over our lifetime and could not be regenerated, period. As it turns out, that's just not true!

With fancy words like neurogenesis and neuroplasticity, scientists are now saying that we can influence the health of our brain, giving us a potentially unlimited ability to change throughout our entire lifespan[1]. That means the better I take care of my brain, the better my brain will take care of me.

My philosophy for mental fitness is based on four simple ideas: feed my brain, rest my brain, exercise my brain, and rewire my brain.

I feed my brain with a low-carb diet that is full of healthy fats, proteins, and vegetables. I also take supplements designed to support healthy brain function. I rest my brain with sleep and meditation. I strive to get a full 8 hours of peaceful sleep every night. I maintain a healthy sleep ritual by:

- Keeping my bedroom dark and cool

- Not using my phone, computer or television in bed

- Going to bed and waking up at a consistent time every day

- Taking a melatonin supplement designed to aid restful sleep

- Drinking a glass of water during the last hour before bed

I also use a practice of daily meditation to rest my brain. Thousands of years of tradition, along with four decades of brain research, have proven that the brain is transformed by meditation[2]. These are the ways I make meditation a daily practice for me:

1. Meditate first thing in the morning.

To reinforce this behavior, I prepare my coffee machine the night before and do my 15 minutes of meditation while my coffee is brewing each morning.

2. Use helpful resources.

I personally like to use Headspace, a digital health platform that provides guided meditation training for its users. During the 10-day free trial, the founder of the company, Andy Puddicombe, teaches the basics of meditation.

Puddicombe is a former Buddhist monk and meditation expert. I like the way he teaches and guides me through each session. Through using Headspace, I learned the importance of self-awareness as a foundation to meditation. At the beginning of a new meditation session, Puddicombe instructs me to scan my body (sensation) and mind (emotion) to see how I feel at the moment, and then to consider why I decided to sit and meditate (intention).

Practicing this "sensation, emotion, and intention" technique has helped bring self-awareness to any task I am involved in, at any time during the day.

3. Measure for consistency.

When I measure something, I focus my attention on it. Headspace supports this best practice by automatically tracking the number of days I have meditated since beginning the program. It also keeps track of "run streaks" which are the number of days I have meditated in a row.

4. Embrace the power of community.

Turning a new behavior into a habit is easier when you share the experience with others. Headspace makes it easy to add a buddy to your meditation group and shows you how many people are meditating throughout the Headspace community.

5. Relax and let go.

I can become embarrassed when I think about how others might judge my meditation practice. I overcome this obstacle by focusing on how important meditation is to me. I just let go of any feelings of embarrassment and sit anyways. Another obstacle I often face is the frustration I feel about my wandering mind. I overcome this challenge by acknowledging that meditating each day is way more important than doing it the "right" way. When my mind wanders I just relax into the feeling and bring my attention back to the moment – without judging the session or myself.

6. If meditation is a priority, then I must meditate.

I heard somewhere that it takes 21 days to form a habit. I do not know if that is fact or myth, but the more I do something, the easier it gets. At some point, it becomes a part of my normal routine. The more I meditate, the more natural it becomes.

I exercise my brain by working out and reading.

It turns out that my practice of lifelong exercise is good for my brain. Scientists now know that exercise promotes the process of neurogenesis, which is your brain's ability to adapt and grow new brain cells, regardless of your age[3].

My daily practice of reading provides mental stimulation to keep my brain strong, alert, and healthy. Studies have shown that staying mentally engaged can slow the progress of (and possibly even prevent)

Alzheimer's and dementia[4].

The fourth and final piece of my philosophy on mental fitness is embracing my power to rewire my brain.

According to Dr. Hilary Stokes, when you repeatedly align your beliefs, feelings and actions, you will experience lasting changes in your brain[5].

Reflection is my practice for cultivating the inner being that is my unique soul. It is a mindfulness practice that helps me slow down, quiet my mind and listen to my heart. It helps me know who I am and what is important to me. Reflection helps me to know what I love and why I love it. I call the things I love doing my "ings":

> Loving, learning, exercising, reading, writing, cooking, meditating, thinking, boating, giving, playing, traveling, entertaining, speaking, researching, and networking.

I am motivated to take excellent care of my brain because I want my brain to take excellent care of me. Happiness and mastery are two key elements that are important to how I care for, and rewire, my brain.

> Happiness: The more I do the things I love, the happier I am.

> Mastery: The more I do the things I love, the closer I get to mastery of them.

Dr. Ellen Domm explains why aligning your beliefs, feelings and actions, as I do with my practice of reflection, is so important. She says "the phrase, 'neurons that fire together wire together,'" is a simplistic way of explaining that "each experience we encounter, including our feelings, thoughts, sensations, and muscle actions becomes embedded in the network of brain cells, that produce that experience. Each time you repeat a particular thought or action, you strengthen the connection between a set of brain cells or neurons."[6]

Incredibly, this means, the more I do the things I love, the more I'm rewiring my brain to love the things I do, and this in turn creates more emotional wellbeing and happiness.

Chapter 9 – My Philosophy for Financial Fitness and Lifelong Work

After physical fitness and mental fitness comes an element to life that some people love and others loathe: financial fitness. My passion for lifelong work is at the core of this next philosophy.

> "There's plenty of money out there. They print more every day." (Grandpa George in *Charlie and the Chocolate Factory*, by Roald Dahl)

I define financial fitness as having the means to provide for yourself and others. Personally, my financial fitness is connected to a deep-seated sense of responsibility to provide for myself and my family. Good financial fitness creates the freedom to do the things we want to do, and to enjoy them to the fullest, without worrying about whether we can truly afford them.

My financial philosophy has four components: engine, purpose, beliefs, and mechanics.

Work is the engine. The Oxford Dictionary defines work as, "activity involving mental or physical effort done in order to achieve a result."[7] I have been working since I was 10 years old, and in that time have been a paperboy, janitor, grocery clerk, sprinkler installer, bartender, retail buyer, sales representative, financial auditor, business executive, entrepreneur, keynote speaker, and author. That's a wide variety of roles, each with its own joys and challenges.

I believe humans are designed to engage in meaningful work. It is a foundational element of health. Work not only feeds my family, it feeds my soul, and makes me happy. I intend to work for the rest of my life.

The purpose of financial fitness is different for everyone and it can change over a lifetime. A person's financial purpose tends to parallel Maslow's hierarchy of needs[8], which means that the purpose of work is first focused on providing basic needs like food and shelter. Once these needs are met and resources grow, one's purpose can expand to creating things of personal value and significance, such as creative pursuits or philanthropic efforts. Along the way, interests, hobbies, stage of life, and responsibilities may influence one's financial purpose.

When I was young, my purpose for work was to earn extra spending money. When I became a family man, my purpose was to provide for my family. Now, my purpose is to create the financial freedom to do the things my wife and I want to do – that is, to live comfortably, enjoy our family and friends, travel the globe, and of course, improve the health and wellbeing of the world, one person at a time through my company, Happy Living.

Personal beliefs about money can be an asset or a liability when it comes to financial fitness. Many people have learned to fear, or be suspicious of, money. Preconceived notions, confusion, and perceptions about finances can have an impact on your earning potential and relationship with money. Here are the beliefs I have about money.

- Be patient, but disciplined. Building wealth is a marathon, not a sprint.

- Give what you can, when you can. Sharing your talents, time and resources creates a powerful positive energy in your life.

- There is an abundance of wealth in the world. Certainly enough for you to have all that you want.

- Specialize and delegate. Spend time on your career and things that bring you joy. Hire professionals to help with household work and other personal services whenever you can, and be willing to delegate at work.

- Be a role model. Demonstrate that money is good by using your money for good.

- Be proud. Build financial success without arrogance and without apology.

I have worked for more than forty years now. There are times when I have worked very hard and other times when I have been able to work smart. In both cases, I've had excellent results and disappointing results. Through the years, though, I have learned that certain processes and attributes generally lead to success.

Below, I have outlined the mechanics I follow for financial fitness as a businessman and an entrepreneur. If you are a teacher or doctor, executive or diplomat, your approach to financial fitness might look very different. The right approach to financial fitness will be unique and personalized to your personality, responsibilities, life, and circumstance. So do your research, listen to your inner wisdom, and find what works for you.

Generating Income

- Find work you want to do for your entire life

- Find work with results that can be broadcast to the world. Try to avoid work with limited geographical reach

- Find work with highly recurring revenue – this means customers pay for the products or services, every month or every year, forever

- Find work with near-zero marginal cost revenue – this means creating a product or a service once, and selling it over and over again

Building Wealth

- Pay yourself first by investing 10% of your income for the future

- Use the discipline of a budget to make certain you are spending less than you are earning

- Invest in home ownership

- Invest in business ownership

Protecting Wealth

- Use insurance wherever possible to reduce the financial impact of unforeseen accidents and disasters

-
- Use annuities to create reliable, long-term future income

I have not come to this knowledge through experience and internal wisdom alone. Many wise people have shared their financial advice, philosophies, victories and failures with me. Some of these people have been the authors of influential books that have impacted my financial philosophy:

- *The Richest Man in Babylon* by George S. Clason

- *Rich Dad Poor Dad* by Robert T. Kiyosaki

- *Die Broke* by Stephen Pollan

Chapter 10 – My Philosophy for Spirituality

The final of the four fitnesses is spiritual fitness. Like all of these philosophies, spirituality is very personal. My philosophy for spirituality focuses on what I refer to as "magnificence." My philosophy might resonate with you, or you might have another way to define your connection to that constant, loving, peaceful presence that is referred to as God, the divine, source energy, oneness, the Universe, and so on.

> "The two most important days in your life are the day you are born and the day you find out why."
> (Mark Twain)

Many years ago when I watched the movie *The Secret* for the first time, I was instantly attracted to a quote from it, "I am magnificence in human form." While the phrase was inspiring, I was also intimidated. The word "magnificence" felt like too grand of a description for me – indeed, almost boastful and arrogant. But "I am magnificence in human form" stuck with me long after I finished watching the movie. It resonated deeply... my attraction to the quote seemed important and worth reflecting on further.

After years of contemplation, reading many books, and taking hundreds of long hikes, the phrase, "I am magnificence in human form," has become the centerpiece of my philosophy on spirituality.

Since I enjoy reading about personal development and spirituality, I have come across many books that have influenced my spiritual philosophy. A few of my favorites include:

The Untethered Soul by Michael A. Singer

Change Your Thoughts – Change Your Life by Dr. Wayne W. Dyer

The Power of Now by Eckhart Tolle

The War of Art by Steven Pressfield

Halftime by Bob Buford

I define spirituality as: discovering and cultivating the inner being that is my unique soul. Spirituality is learning to detect the differences between energy and ideas created by my mind and those generated from deep within my awareness. Spirituality is knowing that my inner spirit is my direct connection to the greater magnificence of everything in the universe.

My spiritual practice is based on slowing down, being quiet, and listening to my heart instead of my head.

This heart-based way of living connects me to my spiritual source. Listening to my heart brings me energy and a sense of ease. When I live from my heart I see abundance everywhere and I feel generous and grateful. In contrast, the head-based way of living connects me to the selfishness of my ego. Listening to my head brings me insecurity, worry, and shame. When I live from my head, I am seeing through the survival-based lens of the human mind, with its scarcity mentality. In that state, I have no access to my experience of the divine and instead feel a need to protect what's mine.

My spiritual practice is to recognize head-based thoughts and actions, and then replace them with heart-based ones. When I do this, joy and grace flows into my life.

Reading Michael A. Singer's book *The Untethered Soul* helped me understand why the heart-based way fuels happiness and spiritual connection. Using the analogy of a pendulum, Singer explains how the ego or mind-based path creates unproductive energy that pushes and pulls from one extreme to the other. Unhelpful thoughts, poor choices, and negativity create energy that forces the pendulum off-center. For example, breaking your diet one day, then feeling guilty and starving yourself the next. Telling a lie to gain something today, then getting caught and suffering the consequences tomorrow. Skipping exercise one day, then going twice as hard the next day and causing an injury. Every push in one direction creates energy of equal force that swings back in the other direction. My pendulum sways off-center when I listen to the selfishness of my mind instead of the wisdom of my heart... and that does not feel good.

There is no swinging from side to side on the heart-based path. Energy is not wasted recovering from bad thoughts or poor choices. The pendulum stops swinging and energy moves forward. This is why I have more energy when I follow my heart. My pendulum comes to rest at the center where there is no energy pushing me in one direction or pulling me the other.

I stay on-center when I listen to my heart and connect to something greater. When I am on-center and in alignment with my beliefs, I feel energy, ease, joy, and grace. When I am on-center, I get into "the zone" as my most creative self — immersed in an interesting project, losing track of time, and performing with ease. Sometimes this alignment manifests as a powerful feeling of gratitude when I'm hiking alone in the natural beauty of wilderness. Other times I find that when I meditate, a wave of beautiful emotion washes over me as I feel a deep connection to the world around me.

When I am on-center and listening to my heart, I am living from the inner spirit that is my unique soul. I recognize and release energy or ideas created by my ego, and instead focus on those generated from within my deeper awareness. When I am on-center, I allow more of my connection with the greater power of the universe. When I am on-center, I have incredible energy, my days are easy, and my life is full of joy. When I am on-center and living by my philosophy on spirituality, I am magnificence in human form… and that feels great.

Chapter 11 – My Philosophy for Love

Following the four fitnesses are the next two Foundations of Health at the middle of the pyramid, love and adventure. In my philosophy for love I examine the various types of love, along with the purpose and power of love in my life.

> "Love is like the wind, you can't see it but you can feel it."
> (Nicholas Sparks)

Love is one of the most powerful forces on earth. Love enables people to follow their dreams against all odds. Love gives us the inner strength to work through terrible events. Love is the mighty glue that binds a couple as they build and share a life together. I believe love is what gives meaning and purpose to life.

So, how can I tell when it's love that I'm feeling? Well, I recognize love when something touches my heart and I can feel it reach my inner spirit. And I look for love everywhere, all the time, by paying attention to what I am attracted to. When I find love, I give it all I have to give. I work to create a life where I do the things I love, with the people I love, in the places I love, from a basis of self-love. My philosophy on love is built on five simple ideas, outlined below.

Self-Love

This is the work I do to be strong, healthy, and happy enough to care for myself, my family, and others. At first glance, it may seem arrogant or egotistical to put this first, but without self-love, any other kind of love cannot flow freely in your life. Love of self gives me the power to contribute to my community. I express love of self when I am living in the moment, listening to my feelings and acting from my heart, and creating my absolute best life by working, learning, exercising, cooking, meditating, thinking, and communing with nature.

Romantic Love

For me, this is a strong and content love with my soul mate. It is a very deep connection that cannot be explained easily. It is a comfort and acceptance I had not experienced until I finally found my beautiful wife.

This love is magical and I'm appreciative of its presence in my life every single day.

Love of Family and Friends

My love of family is best described by the pure love I felt the first time I held a child of my own, as well as the "no matter what" love I feel for my brothers and sister. In addition to my family, I am lucky to have a few friends whom I truly love. These are different and richer than more surface friendships because, for some reason, we match each other somewhere deep within our hearts. These types of friends are another form of soul mate. Finally, my pets (especially dogs) give me a kind of love that just feels good. It is hard to find words to express the love of pets, but the unconditional bond between a pet and its owner is something magical.

Love of Doing

Beyond the love of self, romantic love, and love of others, I have found that there is also a love of doing. A person is expressing this kind of love when they say, "I love what I do." I love working, especially when I am engaged in creative work, producing something that makes a contribution to society, and doing so in connection with my family, friends and community. For me, working includes reading, learning, experimenting and writing about things that improve the health and wellbeing of the world, one person at a time.

I also love playing… this includes exercising, cooking, entertaining, traveling, boating, and paddle boarding. When I am doing any of these things, it is very easy for me to say that I love what I do!

Love of Places

There are certain places that touch my heart whenever I visit, or even just think of them. New York City inspires me. The bustling streets, the energy of the people, the towering skyscrapers, and the tranquility of Central Park all touch something deep inside me. I love visiting New York for business and have also made a point of traveling there for pleasure. It is a magical city that I love.

Sedona, Arizona is another location that has a very special place in my heart. Sedona is a world-renowned travel destination known for its spectacular landscape. It is one of my favorite places on earth and is an anchor for many wonderful memories. My wife introduced me to Sedona on the first weekend we met. It was very romantic and we held hands for two entire days. I remember a complete stranger asking to take our picture as we were gazing at the amazing views. She said she wanted to do this because she "had never seen a couple so in love." I keep that picture in my office and feel a huge burst of love every time I look at it. Sedona is where we got married and hosted our rehearsal dinner. As we said our vows, we could see the iconic ridges of Snoopy Rock. Our wedding weekend was one of the best and most memorable celebrations of love in my life. Sedona is also where my wife and I started buying artwork together and where we hosted an annual Mother's Day brunch for our moms. It is where we escaped for romantic getaways at one of our favorite hotels in the world, L'Auberge de Sedona. It's also a place where I went on many amazing hikes and where my daughter and I hosted a memorable event for Happy Living. My memories of Sedona – all the people I have been there with, the experiences, and natural beauty – have become a deep and permanent part of who I am.

I also love the lake house my wife and I purchased last summer. We choose our home based on schools, its convenient location to the town and airport, and the gorgeous property. The long driveway winds down to a private lakefront retreat. The house is nestled on a picturesque waterfront lot, just under two acres with more than two hundred trees, and 454 feet of shoreline. The lake can be seen from nearly every window in the house with a spectacular 180-degree water view. It's almost impossible to see a road.

The house itself wasn't our favorite, but it was a good size and shape. It was situated well on the property. It had enough to work with. All the things we didn't love could be fixed. We have remodeled it into our dream home that is designed for dual purposes. First, it is a comfortable home for us to live and raise our children. Second, it is our place for celebrating life and love with our family and friends.

Love is a powerful force indeed. Love is many things and takes many forms. Love is different for everyone and it changes over one's lifetime. Love can sometimes feel very complicated, but my philosophy on love is quite simple: I believe love is what gives meaning and purpose to my life – so, for as long as I live, I will keep creating a life doing the things I love, with the people and creatures I love, in the places I love.

Chapter 12 – My Philosophy for Adventure

My philosophy for adventure has two parts: unknown outcomes and continuous exploration. As you will read, I believe in a wide range of adventure – from the adrenaline rush of adventure sports, to the calm excitement of lifelong learning. It is through adventure that I make advances in my pursuit of continuous improvement, and I intend to do so every day for the rest of my life.

Unknown Outcomes

"That which does not kill us makes us stronger."
(Friedrich Nietzsche)

Discovery is thrilling. Learning is rewarding. Creating is fulfilling. Becoming more is invigorating. I feel most alive when I am testing my limits, stepping into something unknown, and beginning another adventure.

Each new day brings another trail to hike, book to read, person to meet, relationship to strengthen, recipe to cook, or idea to investigate. The more I explore "out there" in the world, the more I develop "in here" within myself. Every adventure expands my horizons, inspires me to become more, and nurtures my soul.

I know I am embarking on an adventure when one or more of the following are present:

- There is an element of risk or danger

- I'm trying something new that I've never done before

- The outcome is unknown or unexpected

As you read in the quote above, according to the German philosopher, Friedrich Nietzsche, what doesn't kill you makes you stronger. I put his theory to the test in the summer of 2007 during my fourth annual boys-only rafting trip, when one of my adventures became a near-death experience.

The trip began in the same way as many of my other rafting experiences: I was floating solo down the Cataract Canyon in my own two-person inflatable raft. Our group was nearing a landing beach on the left side of the Colorado River before the three most notorious rapids in the canyon, simply named Big Drop 1, Big Drop 2, and Big Drop 3.

I have always loved the rush of riding rapids and was happy to be out on the river "on my own." But, before I knew what was happening, a wave caught me from the right, slammed me out of my raft, and pushed me towards the bottom of the river. Suddenly, I was struggling to get to the surface, couldn't find which way was up, and started to worry that I would run out of breath. Then I remembered our guide Johnny's advice, "If you're under water and can't find the surface, stop struggling, curl into a ball, and let your life jacket do its job."

I was still tumbling under the water and unable to find the surface. And then I clearly remember thinking, "I hope Johnny is right!" as I curled into a ball as instructed, fighting to keep calm. I quickly popped up to the surface near my son and his fellow rafter. I climbed back into my raft just in time for my son to hand me my paddle, which he'd managed to recover, with a huge grin of relief on his face.

I was worn out from what has just happened, but had to start paddling hard to make it to the beach. Big Drop 1 was roaring just ahead and if I couldn't get there I was going over Big Drops 1, 2, and 3. Alone. I paddled and paddled and paddled. It took every bit of energy I could muster to make it to that beach. When I finally reached the shore, I fell to the ground in a heap of exhaustion and exhilaration.

There is always a considerable risk in taking a rafting trip like the one I just described. However, the reward has been just as worthwhile. Whenever I think of adventure, activities with a real element of danger such as rafting are what first come to mind. The challenge is electrifying. Time slows. Senses heighten. Overcoming unforeseen obstacles is inspiring. Recalling the highs and lows is humbling. The memory lasts forever. Adventure ignites the human spirit, reveals hidden capabilities that lie within us and helps us become more.

Experiences like this have changed me as a person. It seems the bigger the danger and the higher the risk, the more capacity an adventure has to change you. I imagine this is why people try to climb deadly mountains like K2 or Mount Everest. Just to reiterate, though, adventure is all about following your heart, not a prescribed formula. Everyone has a different take – a commitment to a person or task could be a big adventure, just as facing situations you find frightening may be too. Let your excitement about an idea be your indicator, once measured against your priorities, of course. You might feel thrilled (and nervous or scared) by signing up for a marathon or going camping in the wilderness alone. Your definition of adventure is entirely personal and unique to you.

Life is a non-stop opportunity for learning, creating, and becoming more. I believe a better self is always possible today, every day, as long as I keep exploring. Adventure is the primary means of my continuous goal to be more true to my heart and let more of my spirit shine out in this life.

Continuous Exploration

"Security is mostly a superstition. It does not exist in nature, nor do the children of men as a whole experience it. Avoiding danger is no safer in the long run than outright exposure. Life is either a daring adventure, or nothing."
(Helen Keller)

While dangerous adventures have helped shaped my life, there are two other forms of adventure that help me become all that I can be — a lifetime of learning and a persistent willingness to step into the unknown.

I have made a commitment to lifelong learning that provides me with daily opportunities for adventure. Wondering what I might learn next creates a sense of excitement and vitality within me. There are four main ways I pursue lifelong learning: reading, traveling, pursuing hobbies, and trying new experiments for my company, Happy Living.

1. Reading

Reading gives me a quiet and relaxing way to explore the world beyond my own experiences. While there are many reasons to pick up a good book, I mostly read for self-discovery. The books I gravitate towards help me learn from the wisdom of others so that I can better understand myself. Reflecting on what I read helps me organize my thoughts and feelings and bring my newfound understandings into the philosophies that guide my life.

2. Travel

Traveling provides the opportunity to explore the world directly. I have traveled all across America and to twenty other countries. Traveling makes me aware of the size and majesty of our world and my humble place within it. Each trip is an opportunity to discover new places, cultures, foods, and ideas. When I am able, I enjoy sharing those experiences with people I love, my family and friends.

3. Hobbies

Hobbies give me an opportunity to play with new ideas, toys and experiences. When my wife and I moved to our lake house, I decided to dedicate my recreational time to playing on the water. Swimming, paddle boarding and boating are hobbies that connect me with nature and adventure. I have also taken on cooking as a hobby, which helps me enjoy my philosophy for good nutrition even more.

4. Experiments

"Happy Living Experiments" are the research and resources I explore so that I can help improve the wellbeing of the world, one person at a time. Whether it's trying to learn how to reduce the number of harmful chemicals in my household, or figuring out how to align my fitness practices with my lifestyle goals, every experiment is an opportunity for better health and happiness.

My commitment to self-improvement has become a way of life. Improvement requires change, change invites risk, and risk creates fear of failure, embarrassment, losing money or friends, or even worse. As I mentioned earlier, the risk involved in dangerous adventures can even be life threatening. Overcoming fear requires the courage to venture into a land of unknown outcomes. Deciding to act in spite of uncertainty is how one's life becomes a daring adventure.

Cultivating a persistent willingness to say, "YES!" to change has led me on incredible adventures that I never could have imagined. Walking into the land of unknown outcomes has taken me on a wild ride, including working ten different jobs, living in more than ten houses in seven states, owning four businesses, moving cross-country four times, raising two children, marrying, divorcing, marrying again, and raising two more children. Although I never ended up exactly where I expected, each adventure enriched my life. Each step into the unknown helped me become more than I was before.

Erik Weihenmayer, the first blind person to summit Mount Everest, is an inspiration and a true adventurer. In an interview with Oprah's TV network OWN, he said, "Sometimes that fear of reaching out into the unknown paralyzes people to the point they decide not to reach out at all. For me, all the great things that have ever come to me have come through reaching out into that unknown."

In 18 words, Erik captured the essence of my philosophy on adventure: all the great things that have ever come to me have come through reaching out into that unknown.

It doesn't matter how fast I go, it only matters that I remain willing to explore the people, places, ideas and things that flow into my life.

Chapter 13 – My Philosophy for Significance

The pinnacle of the Seven Foundations of Health is significance. In my philosophy for significance I share what this concept means to me and why "leaving a mark" is a key to cultivating a meaningful life.

> "Success is winning. Significance is helping others win. Success leaves a fingerprint on creation. Significance leaves a footprint on the soul."
> (D. Trinidad Hunt)

Significance sits alone atop the pyramid of the Seven Foundations of Health because I believe it's what the game is all about – leaving an exclamation mark on a life! My philosophy on significance has two components: doing something you love and creating something of value to others.

Significance is doing something that is inspired by love. For example, let's say I have a lot of money and my accountant suggests I could get a tax break if I give a $1 million donation to help underprivileged children. Is that significant? Not in my book. While it's true I would be giving something of value to others, it would be for personal gain, not inspired by love. And that doesn't mean the opposite is simply to not give at all, but to find something that holds real significance for you. Suppose that in another situation, I don't have a lot of extra money or time, but I love working with kids. In this scenario, I volunteer 5 hours a week at a local school. Is that significant? Yes! I am doing what I love and creating something of value to others too.

As you can see from the examples above, I have the chance to create something significant when the actions I take are in alignment with who I am on a spiritual level. When this is the case, doing what I love does not feel like work at all. Instead, it feels important. It feels connected to something more. It feels right. In the end, significance is doing, inspired by love.

Significance can also be defined as creating something of value for the benefit of others. Imagine that I love to compose music and play the piano. I love playing the piano so much that I play incredible music every day in a soundproof room, all by myself. Is that significant? Not according to me. While I would be doing something I love, I am not creating anything of value to others. Let's change the story, just a bit. I love to compose music and play the piano. I play every day in a soundproof room, by myself, making incredible recordings that bring people joy. Is that significant? Yes! I am creating something of value to others through the process of doing what I love.

I have the chance to create something significant when the actions I take serve others. Doing work becomes meaningful when it serves others. It feels important. It feels connected to something more. It resonates with your heart and feels right.

We have an interview series on the Happy Living blog called Something Significant, which showcases ordinary people doing extraordinary things. Each interview highlights a person immersed in work they love, creating something deeply connected to who they are, and bringing value to others.

We have interviewed Dr. Tom Sult, who's focus has been in the field of changing how doctors treat patients, and Elise Cripe, an entrepreneur and mother of two, who turned her love for "getting things done" into a business. We shared James FitzGerald's story about how he went from being named The Fittest on Earth at the inaugural CrossFit Games in 2007 to optimizing personal fitness through his business, OPEX Fitness. We were inspired by Nick Black, a veteran who after his service went on to earn his MBA and start the nonprofit, Stop Soldier Suicide. There are countless stories of people just like you and me, who have found a way to do what they love while giving back and creating something of value to others. I invite you to take some time to explore the interviews – I'm sure they'll fill you with insight and inspiration.

I would like to return for a moment to the topic of reflection. I use my practice of reflection to keep my focus on what is most important to me and to stay connected to what I love. Reflection helps me slow down, quiet my mind, and listen to my heart. It helps me know who I am on a spiritual level. Reflection helps me to know what is important to me, what I love and why.

One great result that has come out of my practice of reflection is what I call "The Seven Wonders of My Life." Keeping these in mind and thinking of them often keeps me connected to my true self and in a state of gratitude for all the joy and happiness in my life. I'm honored to share them with you here.

The Seven Wonders of My Life are:

- One True Love: being a loving and devoted husband

- Family: providing love, support, and leadership

- Friends: connecting and celebrating life together

- Fitness: caring for my body, mind, and spirit

- Finance: investing in charities, businesses, and people doing good work

- Adventure: exploring different places, new experiences, and fresh ideas

- Business: researching, experimenting, and writing about best practices for happy living

When I prioritize my time, energy, and resources on these Seven Wonders, I increase my chances of doing something significant. Each of these is in deep alignment with who I am. They touch my heart and bring me joy. I practice my philosophy for significance by finding the intersection between what I love and creating value for others. That is what puts the exclamation mark on my life! It is my sincere wish you will be inspired to take the time to reflect on and appreciate the wonderful "wonders" in your life too.

Chapter 14 – My Philosophy for Why We're Here

If significance is the pinnacle of my personal philosophies, then my philosophy for why we're here is its culmination. In this philosophy, I share my personal answers to one of life's biggest questions, "Why are we here?" While it can be challenging to try to define our reason for being, finding my answers to this question has helped me build a robust and helpful Belief Road Map for my life.

> "It's not just what you have, but it's what you do with what you have. Who are you lifting up? Who are you making better?"
> (Denzel Washington)

The goal of my philosophies is to create a Belief Road Map that will help me evolve into the fully realized and optimized person I have the capacity to become. My philosophies inspire me to pursue continuous improvement and help guide me on my path.

Practicing gratitude, paying attention to what inspires me, maintaining order, and doing work that is meaningful are all practices that help me pursue my philosophy for happy living.

Following a diet that reduces inflammation and exercising consistently helps me maintain my physical fitness. Feeding, resting, exercising, and rewiring my brain helps me maintain my mental fitness. Following my financial philosophy helps me generate income, and build and manage wealth.

Slowing down, being quiet, and listening to my heart instead of my head is what keeps me on my spiritual path. Doing the things I love, with the people I love, in the places I love is what gives meaning and purpose to my life. Creating value for others while doing what I love is what gives my life significance.

"Dangerous" adventures and continuous exploration have led me to step into the land of unknown outcomes, where nothing is guaranteed. All of the great things that have ever come to me have come through reaching out into that unknown. Stepping into the unknown of life's adventures is even more meaningful when you consider their exponential power…

Every experience, the good and bad, changes me in some way. Every adventure I survive. Every book I read. Every relationship I develop. Every country I explore. Every new hobby I learn. Every time I start a new job, or get fired from one, or move to a new city, or marry, or divorce, or have children. Each of these things changes me and adds to the network of my total experience. There is a hidden power within my network of knowledge and experience that helps me grow exponentially.

In technology, Metcalfe's Law explains how the value of a physical network grows with the addition of each new device or member. According to Wikipedia, "the law has been often illustrated using the example of fax machines: a single fax machine is useless, but the value of every fax machine increases with the total number of fax machines in the network, because the total number of people with whom each user may send and receive documents increases."[9]

Life experiences work the same way. A single experience may contribute little to the life of a person. But, like the fax machine, the value of every experience increases with the total number of experiences in one's lifetime. Circumstances that you once considered failures may have revealed their true purpose to you, and the invaluable learning you have gained from them is suddenly understood. As each new experience changes you, the value of every past experience, life lesson, or challenge compounds exponentially within the "new" you.

For example, one thing that happens today may create a sudden insight into the true value and meaning of an event from decades before. With each experience, you build an evolving and growing network of knowledge to draw upon. This is why "experienced" people seem so smart – they have tapped into the exponential power of becoming more.

Four concepts help me remain persistently willing to reach out into the unknown, even when the path appears hard, scary, or even impossible to pass. These are:

- I know each step on my path of continuous improvement helps me grow exponentially

- I accept fear as a natural response to the unknown, not an excuse to say NO.

- I say YES to opportunities to learn, grow, explore, and go, even in the face of uncertainty

- I reflect on how my life experiences change who I am and what I want over time

The more I venture into the land of unknown outcomes, the more I become. And the more I become, the more I am able to give. Giving is the ultimate land of unknown outcomes. It is impossible to know how much one simple act of kindness or a helping hand will mean to another person.

"Even if no one sees or acknowledges it," writes Dr. Wayne Dyer in *Change Your Thoughts – Change Your Life*, "a silent blessing or thought of love towards others contains a vibration that will be felt throughout the cosmos." Just like the exponential power within a network of devices and experiences, the exponential power of giving is real. When you give, you are creating ripples of positivity with unlimited potential.

I believe we are here to become all we are capable of becoming with the gifts we are given so that we can give to others, lift them up, and help them become all they are capable of becoming too. The enormous energy of such a virtuous cycle of giving is enough to improve the health and wellbeing of the world, one person at a time. What could be more powerful than that?

Chapter 15 – Using Your Belief Road Map

The purpose of this book is to help you know yourself better, identify your priorities, and use your beliefs to create personal philosophies to guide the way to the life of your dreams. We hope that Matt's sharing of his own experiences and processes will give you the structure, guidance, and inspiration to create your own Belief Road Map.

How to Create Your Belief Road Map

Now that you have a practical, specific sense of how to do this, we would like to take the opportunity to set out the process in full, from beginning to end. Of course, you'll never really be done – because you are a constantly evolving, learning, and growing from every experience! However, the Belief Road Map you create will support and guide you on your journey from this day forward, and it can be updated as you move along your path. So, don't let the mind persuade you to put it off until later. Begin now, and start living the life of your dreams today.

Here we go… *The Belief Road Map* process set out for you. It is our sincere wish that following this brings you joy, health, happiness, and a life full of love, adventure and significance.

Step 1. The Power of Reflection

The process of creating your personal philosophies and Belief Road Map begins with reflection. It is a powerful tool when given the right amount of time and intention. The good news is that reflection is free and it's something you can do anytime and anywhere. While reflection isn't always easy, with enough practice it will become an invaluable process. As Matt mentioned in his philosophy for why we're here, there is an exponential power in experience. This means that with every new experience, there is a new opportunity for building your knowledge of yourself and the world around you through reflection.

Step 2. Priorities Guide the Way

With reflection as the starting point, you have learned that aligning your priorities with your beliefs will guide the way to your dream life. When you are able to minimize the *"shoulds"* in your life, you can focus on what really matters: the things, people, experiences and ideas that touch your heart and are connected to your goals and dreams. Through reflection and defining your priorities, you have begun to uncover your true self – an evolving, powerful, magnificent, and completely unique being.

Step 3. Your Personal Philosophies

We shared Happy Living's Seven Foundations of Health and Matt's philosophies on everything from physical fitness to significance with the intention that they will be helpful resources as you craft your own philosophies.

Your personal philosophies make up the Belief Road Map that will lead you on the path to living your dream life. Take your time in creating and shaping them with your experiences and beliefs. If it feels good and resonates with your heart, it goes in. If not, leave it out for now. Remember, there's no wrong way to cultivate your beliefs, define your priorities, and craft your personal philosophies. This process is all about listening to your heart and using your inner wisdom to create philosophies that are aligned with the real you.

If you get confused or unsure at any point as you create your Belief Road Map, ask yourself how the philosophy you are creating makes you feel. If the answer is excited, joyful, and (maybe) a little bit scared, then you're on the right track. Then do everything in your power to act from your philosophies as you go about daily life. Once you're on your way, make sure to revise and update your philosophies as you learn and grow through life. The concepts and ideas that make up your Belief Road Map are built from who you are at your core; they reflect the meaning and purpose of you. What better way to guide yourself to the life of your dreams than by following the inner wisdom that is within you and only you?

We would like to wish you every success with your journey. We are truly humbled and honored to be part of your path to a happier, richer and more fulfilling life

Notes

[1] Chopra.com: "Rewire Your Brain for Happiness"
<http://www.chopra.com/ccl/rewire-your-brain-for-happiness>

[2] *Super Brain* by Deepak Copra, MD and Rudolph E. Tani, PhD

[3] Mercola.com: "The Remarkable Effects of Exercise on Cognition and Brain Cell Regeneration"
<http://fitness.mercola.com/sites/fitness/archive/2015/01/23/brain-benefits-exercise.aspx>

[4] ABCNews.com: "Reading, Chess May Help Fight Alzheimer's"
<http://abcnews.go.com/Health/story?id=117588>

[5] MindBodyGreen.com: "5 Ways To Rewire Your Brain for Meaningful Life Changes" by Dr. Hilary Stokes
<http://www.mindbodygreen.com/0-11762/5-ways-to-rewire-your-brain-for-meaningful-life-changes.html>

[6] DrDomm.com: "Neurons That Fire Together Wire Together" by Dr. Ellen Domm
< http://www.drdomm.com/neurons-the-fire-together-wire-together/>

[7] OxfordDictionaries.com: "Definition of work in English"
<http://www.oxforddictionaries.com/us/definition/american_english/work>

[8] Psychology.About.com: "Hierarchy of Needs by Kendra Cherry"
<http://psychology.about.com/od/theoriesofpersonality/a/hierarchyneeds.htm>

[9] Wikipedia.org: "Metcalfe's Law"
< https://en.wikipedia.org/wiki/Metcalfe%27s_law>

About the Author

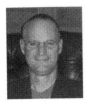

Author. Speaker. Entrepreneur.

On a mission to improve the health and wellbeing of the world, one person at a time.

Founder, HappyLiving.com
Board Member, Fluoresentric.com

Hi, I'm Matt Gersper!

I live on Lake Norman in Mooresville, North Carolina with my beautiful wife and our two daughters.

I graduated from the University of California - Davis where I studied Economics, ran track, and played football. I dedicated my first two years after college to becoming a professional athlete, only to come up short with the unique distinction of being cut from three different teams, in three different leagues: Canadian, USFL, and NFL.

Over the next 30 years, I focused on training myself to become a successful businessman. I was given many opportunities to learn and gain expertise in the various functions required to start, grow, and lead successful businesses.

I have shifted my focus from helping businesses to helping people. On January 16, 2014, I decided to sell my previous company and dedicate my time and resources to researching and sharing best practices for happy living.

I write to inspire others to believe that a better self is always possible – today, every day, for the rest of their lives.

Other Books by Matt Gersper

Turning Inspiration Into Action: How to connect to the powers you need to conquer negativity, act on the best opportunities, and live the life of your dreams.

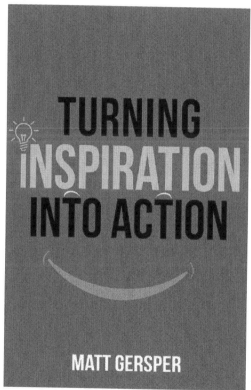

Do you have great ideas that never get done? Do you get inspired and excited one day, and then return to your same old routine the next, without taking action to make your dreams a reality?

Procrastination, self-doubt, cultural expectations, and even the language we use stops so many of us from creating the life we dream about.

Turning Inspiration into Action reveals a time-tested, easy to understand process that works for anyone desiring a better life. Whether you're young or old, rich or poor, if you struggle to turn your big ideas into reality, this book is for you.

Matt Gersper believes that every human being has an inner capacity that is often untapped and truly astonishing in its power. He uses a surprisingly simple process designed to access that inner power in order to bring big ideas to life.

Join Our Community

Be advised of upcoming books and updates from Happy Living! We are on a mission to improve the health & wellbeing of the world, one person at a time. Our blog is filled with ideas for living with health, abundance, and compassion: www.happyliving.com